Westfield Memorial Library
Westfield, New Jersey

D0936757

Westfield Memorial Library
Westfield, New Jersey

A Grant from

The New Jersey State Library

GETTING STRONGER, GETTING FIT

THE IMPORTANCE OF EXERCISE

Westfield Memorial Library
Westfield, New Jersey

OBESITY & KIDS

Westfield Memorial Library
Westfield, New Jersey

GETTING STRONGER, GETTING FIT

THE IMPORTANCE OF EXERCISE

BY JAMIE HUNT

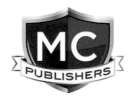

Mason Crest Publishers

Copyright © 2011 by Mason Crest Publishers. All rights reserved. No part of this publication may be reproduced or transmitted in any form or by any means, electronic or mechanical, including photocopying, recording, taping, or any information storage and retrieval system, without permission from the publisher.

MASON CREST PUBLISHERS INC.
370 Reed Road
Broomall, Pennsylvania 19008
(866)MCP-BOOK (toll free)
www.masoncrest.com

First Printing
9 8 7 6 5 4 3 2 1

Library of Congress Cataloging-in-Publication Data

Hunt, Jamie.
  Getting stronger, getting fit : the importance of exercise / by Jamie Hunt.
      p. cm.
  Includes bibliographical references and index.
  ISBN 978-1-4222-1709-2 (hardcover)   ISBN 978-1-4222-1705-4 (series)
  ISBN 978-1-4222-1897-6 (pbk.)   ISBN 978-1-4222-1893-8 (pbk. series)
  1. Exercise—Juvenile literature. 2. Physical fitness—Juvenile literature. I. Title.
  RA781.H796 2010
  613.7—dc22
                                    2010017921

Design by MK Bassett-Harvey and Wendy Arakawa.
Produced by Harding House Publishing Service, Inc.
www.hardinghousepages.com
Cover design by Torque Advertising and Design
Printed in USA by Bang Printing

The creators of this book have made every effort to provide accurate information, but it should not be used as a substitute for the help and services of trained professionals.

CONTENTS

INTRODUCTION FOR THE TEACHERS

We as a society often reserve our harshest criticism for those conditions we understand the least. Such is the case for obesity. Obesity is a chronic and often-fatal disease that accounts for 400,000 deaths each year. It is second only to smoking as a cause of premature death in the United States. People suffering from obesity need understanding, support, and medical assistance. Yet what they often receive is scorn.

Today, children are the fastest growing segment of the obese population in the United States. This constitutes a public health crisis of enormous proportions. Living with childhood obesity affects self-esteem, which down the road can affect employment and attainment of higher education. But childhood obesity is much more than a social stigma. It has serious health consequences.

Childhood obesity increases the risk for poor health in adulthood—but also even during childhood. Depression, diabetes, asthma, gallstones, orthopedic diseases, and other obesity-related conditions are all on the rise in children. Recent estimates suggest that 30 to 50 percent of children born in 2000 will develop type 2 diabetes mellitus, a leading cause of preventable blindness, kidney failure, heart disease, stroke, and amputations. Obesity is undoubtedly the most pressing nutritional disorder among young people today.

If we are to reverse obesity's current trend, there must be family, community, and national objectives promoting healthy eating and exercise. As a nation, we must demand broad-based public-health initiatives to limit TV watching, curtail junk food advertising toward children, and promote physical activity. More than rhetoric, these need to be our rallying cry. Anything short of this will eventually fail, and within our lifetime obesity will become the leading cause of death in the United States if not in the world. This series is an excellent first step in battling the obesity crisis by educating young children about the risks, the realities, and what they can do to build healthy lifestyles right now.

CHAPTER 1 AN OVERWEIGHT WORLD

Did you know that people all over the globe are getting fatter? There are more than 1 billion adults around the world who are **overweight**. At least 300 million of them are **obese**.

But it's not just grownups who are overweight and obese. More and more children are overweight too, even very young children. Around the world, at least 42 million children who are younger than five are overweight.

What's the difference between being overweight and being obese? Both words mean that a person has too much body fat, so much so that it's a health risk. But a person who is obese has much more fat than a person who is overweight, and the health risks are greater as well.

Obesity Around the World

Female

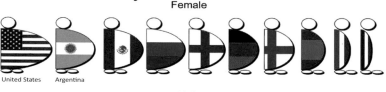

Male

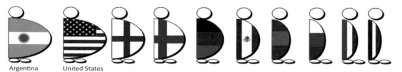

Obesity is a worldwide problem. Using flags to show different countries, this image shows the growing size of both men and women all around the world.

HOW DO YOU KNOW IF YOU'RE OVERWEIGHT?

Experts have figured out a way to help you know if you are in the healthy weight range for your height. It's called the body mass index or BMI. The BMI formula uses height and weight to come up with a BMI number. Though the formula is the same for adults and children, figuring out what the BMI number means is a little more complicated for kids. For children, BMI is plotted on a growth chart that tells whether a child is underweight, healthy weight, overweight, or obese. Different BMI charts are used for boys and girls who are younger than twenty, because the amount of body fat differs between boys and girls. Also, the amount of body fat that is healthy is different, depending on whether you're a toddler or a teenager.

DID YOU KNOW?

In the United States, 15 percent of all children between the ages of 6 and 11 are overweight. That means that if you have 100 children in a room, chances are 15 of them would be overweight. Next, if you were to put 100 kids who were between the ages of 12 and 19 all in one room, you'd be likely to find that 18 of them (18 percent) would be overweight. And if you then put 100 grown-ups together, 67 of them would be overweight or obese. That's more than two-thirds of all grownups!

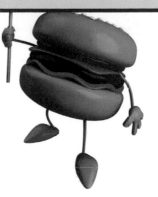

Each BMI chart is divided into percentiles. A child whose BMI is equal to or greater than the 5th percentile and less than the 85th percentile is considered a healthy weight for his or her age. A child at or above the 85th percentile but less than the 95th percentile for age is considered overweight. A child at or above

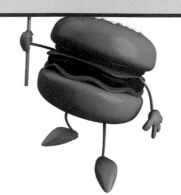

DID YOU KNOW?

Smoking is the number-one cause of deaths that could be prevented. Obesity is the number-two cause of all deaths that could otherwise have been prevented.

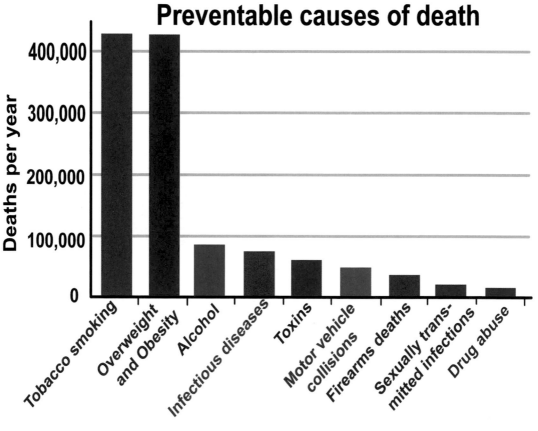

Preventable causes of death

Deaths per year

- 400,000
- 300,000
- 200,000
- 100,000
- 0

Tobacco smoking · Overweight and Obesity · Alcohol · Infectious diseases · Toxins · Motor vehicle collisions · Firearms deaths · Sexually trans-mitted infections · Drug abuse

This chart shows the leading causes of preventable deaths in the United States.

the 95th percentile is considered obese. A child below the 5th percentile is considered underweight.

If you know how much you weigh and how tall you are, you can look at these charts and see for yourself whether you are overweight or obese—but it's also a good idea to talk to your doctor (even if that seems embarrassing). BMI is not always right, so a doctor will be better able to tell you if your weight is healthy or not.

THE DANGERS OF BEING OBESE OR OVERWEIGHT

So what's so bad about being overweight or obese? People come in all different sizes and shapes—and no one should ever be insulted or treated with less respect because of their weight. People who are over-weight or obese can still be smart and pretty and funny. But being overweight can be dangerous. It puts you at risk for getting sick, both now, when you're still a kid, and later, when you grow up.

Children who are overweight or obese are more likely to get diabetes. This is a dis-ease where your body doesn't break down

DID YOU KNOW?

At least 2.6 million people each year die as a result of being overweight or obese.

sugar the way it should. If you have diabetes, you will probably have to take medicine or have special shots every day to help your body process sugar normally. Diabetes can lead to other diseases as well, including blindness. It can make it hard for you to heal after a cut or injury.

DID YOU KNOW?

Being overweight and not exercising enough causes one-third of all cancers.

Being overweight also increases your chances of having heart disease. This is an illness we usually connect with older people, but carrying too much weight around is hard on your heart, no matter how old you are. Even worse, the heavier you are,

Exercise doesn't have to mean going to a gym. Children can get exercise just by playing—and they need about an hour each day.

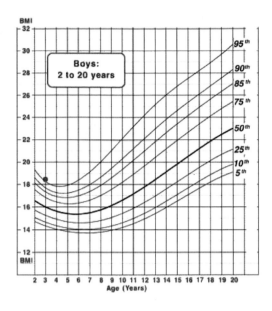

Mike's BMI-for-age falls above the 95th percentile on the BMI-for-age chart for boys so he would be considered overweight.

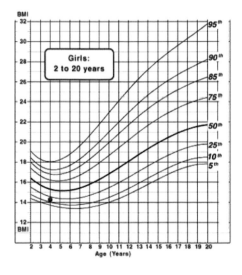

Plotted on the BMI-for-age chart for girls, Mindy's BMI-for-age falls just above the 10th percentile indicating that her BMI is within normal range.

BMI-for-age charts are different for girls and boys, ages 2–20. In this image, the top growth chart shows that a three-year-old boy named Mike, who is 39.7 inches tall (100.8 cm) and weighs 41 pounds (18.6 kg), falls in the 95th percentile. The bottom chart plots the BMI of a four-year-old girl named Mindy. She is 41.9 inches (106.4 cm) and 35.5 pounds (16.1 kg) and the red dot shows that she is in the 10th percentile.

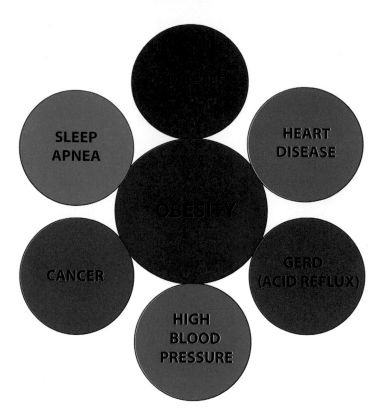

SLEEP APNEA

HEART DISEASE

OBESITY

CANCER

GERD (ACID REFLUX)

HIGH BLOOD PRESSURE

Obesity raises the risk of many illnesses and syndromes, including heart problems and diabetes.

What is cancer? Cancer is a disease that causes the cells in different parts of your body to grow too fast, to the point that they kill healthy cells.

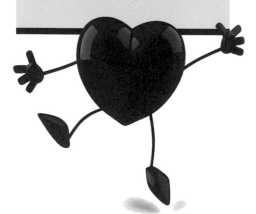

the harder it will probably be for you to run around and exercise. Your heart and lungs need exercise to be healthy. Today, more and more children are obese or overweight—and more and more children are getting heart disease.

Overweight children are also likely to stay that way as they grow up. Being obese or overweight when you are an adult can put you at risk for even more diseases. The extra weight puts strain on your joints, which can lead to arthritis, a disease that makes your joints swollen, stiff, and sore. Obesity may also cause certain kinds of **cancer**.

As people who are overweight or obese grow older, the added weight on their bodies can also lead to other problems, like **high blood pressure** (which increases your chances of having a **stroke**), **gallbladder** disease, and breathing problems. Being overweight can also mean that you have more problems handling your emotions. People who are obese or overweight are more likely to have **depression**.

What does high blood pressure and stroke mean? High blood pressure is when blood pushes against the walls of the blood vessels harder than is normal. This tends to happen when the vessels become too narrow.

A stroke is when the cells in your brain suddenly die because they don't get enough blood.

What is your gallbladder? Your gallbladder is an organ in your body that helps you digest fats.

What is depression? Depression is an emotional illness that makes people feel very sad most of the time.

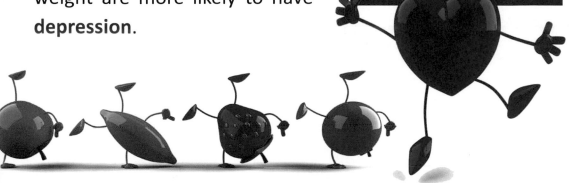

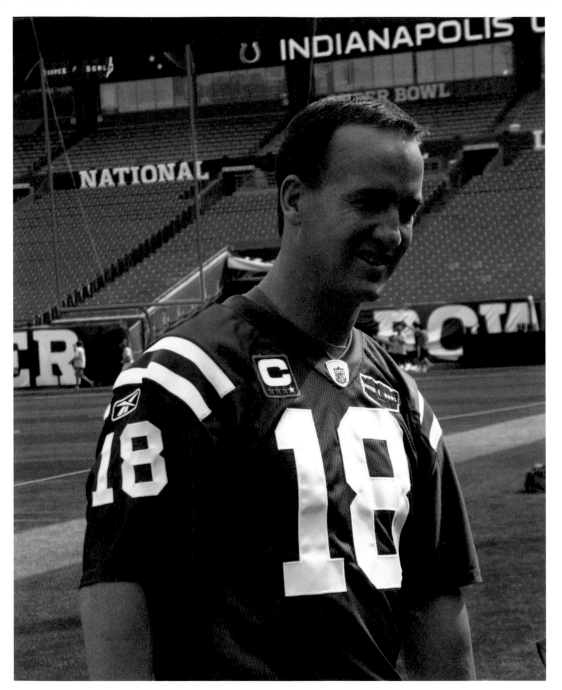

BMI is often not accurate for athletes who have lots of muscle. For example, quarterback Peyton Manning is a fit football player, but with a BMI of 27.3 he is considered overweight.

SO WHY ARE SO MANY PEOPLE OVERWEIGHT?

People don't want to be overweight. In fact, every year around the world people spend millions of dollars on trying NOT to be fat. They buy diet books and diet products; they join gyms and buy exercise equipment. And yet something's not working. More and more people keep getting fatter.

Obesity has many causes. But a huge reason for the world's obesity is our modern lifestyle. We just don't move enough!

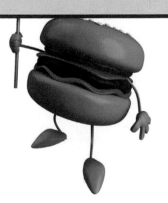

DID YOU KNOW?

Even though doctors use BMI to determine if you're overweight or obese, BMI is sometimes wrong. That's because people who have lots of muscle can also weigh more, even though they don't have much fat.

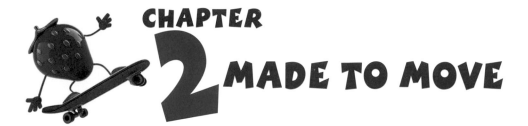

CHAPTER 2 MADE TO MOVE

Your body was made to move. Your muscles are designed to **expand** and **contract**, pulling your bones and bending your joints. Thousands of years ago, our ancestors spent their entire days walking, running, climbing,

What does expand and contract mean? It means to get loose and then pull tight.

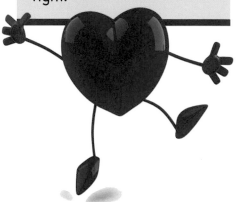

Ancient people had to do a lot of work—and burn a lot of calories—just to survive.

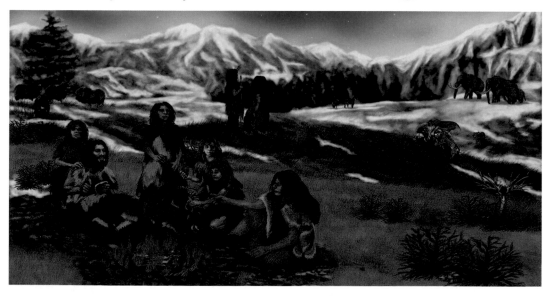

What is energy? Energy is the ability to be active, the power it takes to move.

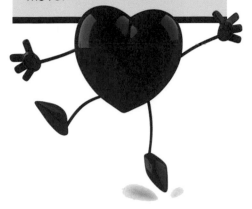

stretching, and throwing. Chasing animals for food, collecting food from plants, fighting off enemies: the effort it took just to survive kept people in better shape back then than most of today's athletes are today.

ENERGY

Moving your body takes **energy**—and your body gets energy from the food you eat. If your body was a car, your food would be the gasoline,

Your calorie needs depend on your age, size, activity level and sex. In general, boys need to eat more calories than girls.

Recommended Daily Calories		
Age	Boys	Girls
2	1000	1000
3	1000–1400	1000–1200
4–5	1200–1400	1200–1400
6	1400–1600	1200–1400
7	1400–1600	1200–1600
8	1400–1600	1400–1600
9	1600–1800	1400–1600
10	1600–1800	1400–1800
11	1800–2000	1600–1800
12	1800–2200	1600–2000
13	2000–2200	1600–2000
14	2000–2400	1800–2000
15	2200–2600	1800–2000
16–18	2400–2800	1800–2000
19–20	2600–2800	2000–2200

DID YOU KNOW?

People who are bigger, more active, or who are growing usually need more calories than smaller people, people who don't move around very much, and people who aren't growing.

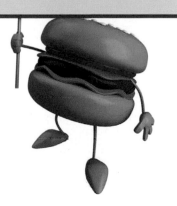

the fuel your body burns to make it "run." All food gives you energy, but some foods give you more than others.

We talk about inches and feet (or centimeters and meters) when we want to measure how long or tall something is; we use pints and quarts (or liters) to measure liquids like milk and soda—and we use calories to measure how much energy is in a certain food.

Each one of us needs a certain amount of calories every day to be healthy and have the energy we need for all the things we do in a day. Even sitting still takes a certain number of calories, but the more active we are, the more calories we need. A car that's sitting in the driveway doesn't need much fuel to keep it running—but a car that's driving fast out on the highway will need much more. Your body is the same.

When we eat more calories than we need, our bodies store the extra energy as fat. Long ago, our ancestors went through times when they had plenty of food, followed by times when food was scarcer. Their bodies' stores of fat helped them get through the times when they had less food. Today, though, many times our bodies just keep storing more and more fat that never needs

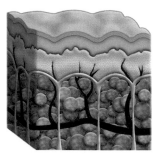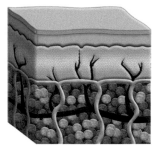

One of the places the human body stores fat is in the deepest layer of skin.

to be used. When that happens, we end up being overweight or obese.

THE TRUTH ABOUT SITTING

DID YOU KNOW?

A recent study found that most children spend nearly 5 hours per day on the computer, watching TV, or playing video games.

Scientists did an experiment with rats and pigs, where they kept the animals still and didn't let them run around. Then the scientists tested the animals to find out what was going on inside their bodies. The scientists discovered that the animals that didn't run around for hours no longer had very much of a chemical called lipase in their bodies. Lipase helps break down fat molecules. Without so much lipase in their bodies, the animals stopped burning calories as fuel—and started getting fat instead.

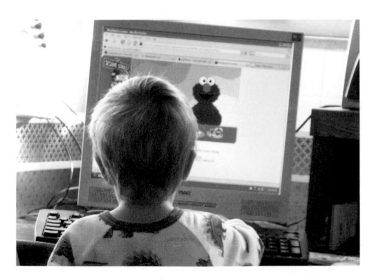

Children begin using computers at a young age—and often spend too much time sitting instead of running and playing.

So the **researchers** decided next to find out what happens to human beings who sit still for long periods of time. They found that not moving around for hours in a row does the same thing to people that it does to rats and pigs—it makes them stop burning calories and start getting fat.

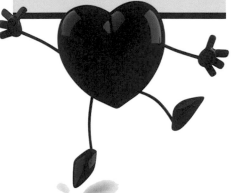

What are researchers? They're people who do experiments and try to find the answers to questions.

Scientists found that rats that sat still too much started getting fat because they no longer had a chemical they needed to break down fat.

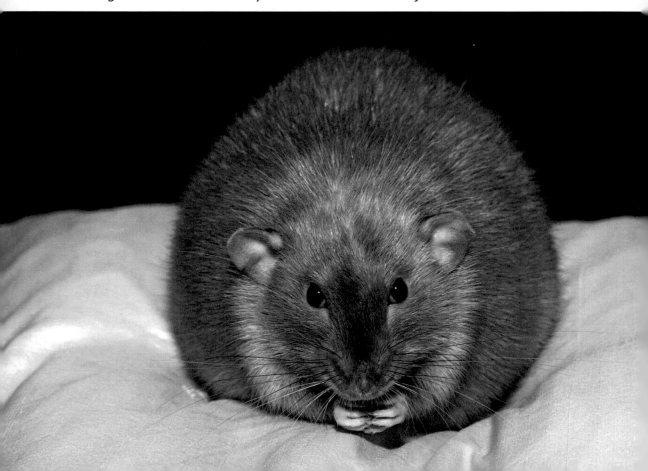

CHANGING LIFESTYLES

A hundred years ago, even fifty years ago, most grownups had plenty of physical work to do that kept them active. Keeping a house clean and growing food took up a lot of time—and burned a lot of calories. Children had chores to do, as well, and when their chores were done, children played games like tag and hide-and-go-seek and hopscotch. All these games involved MOVING. In those days, people moved their bodies every single day.

But that's not the way we live today. Labor-saving inventions like washing machines and vacuum cleaners mean we can keep our homes and clothing clean without working so hard. We buy our food at the grocery store, and often our food comes in quick, easy-to-fix packages—or we eat out at a restaurant. Daily life just doesn't take as much effort as it once did.

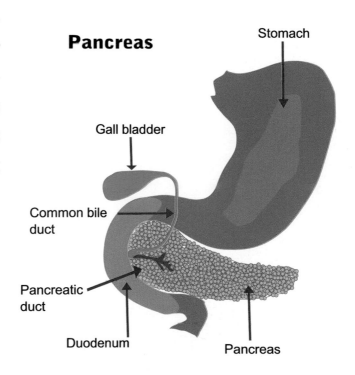

Pancreas

Stomach

Gall bladder

Common bile duct

Pancreatic duct

Duodenum

Pancreas

Lipase, a chemical that helps break down fat, is produced by the pancreas. The pancreas is part of the digestive system.

That seems like a good thing. After all, if we have less work to do, then we have more time to enjoy ourselves. And that would be fine—except the things we do today to enjoy ourselves often don't involve moving our bodies.

Think about what most people do every day. Many grown-ups work in an office where they sit in front of a computer all day. Children go to school, where for much of the day they sit at desks. In the evenings, people come home—and then what do they do? Chances are, they sit down and watch television.

In the past, the games children played, like hopscotch, burned more calories than today's video games and television. Just 30 minutes of hopscotch can burn about 70–80 calories depending on your weight.

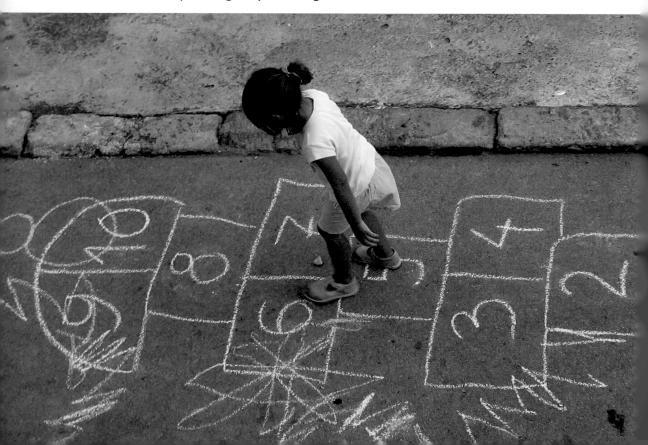

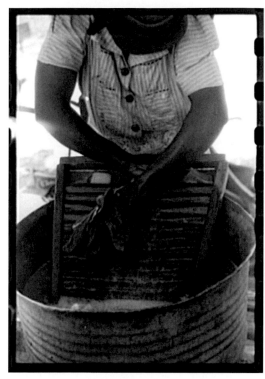

Daily chores like washing the clothes used to take a lot more energy to complete—and burn more calories— than they do today.

They might listen to music on their iPods or MP3 players. Or they sit at their computers and play games or surf the Net.

And then they go to bed, get up the next morning—and spend another day sitting. No wonder so many adults and children are obese or over-weight!

Our bodies were made to move. And when we don't move, we not only gain weight—we also become less healthy in other ways as well.

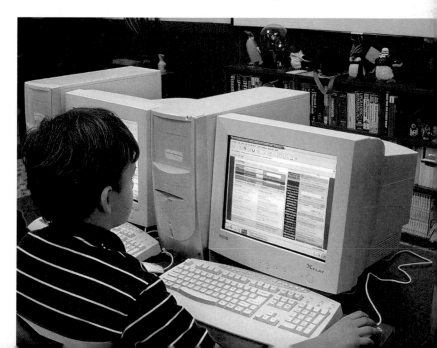

Every day, on average, 8–18 year-olds spend about four hours watching TV, fifty minutes playing video games and over one hour on the computer.

CHAPTER 3
EXERCISE IS GOOD FOR YOU!

Moving around is what your body is made to do. When you exercise regularly, you not only help your body use calories in a healthy way, you also make all the cells and organs in your body healthier. When you're strong and fit, your body makes good use of the food you eat, and all your body parts are much more likely to work together the way they're supposed to. This means that even when you're not exercising, you burn more calories. You feel better, physically and emotionally— and you even think better!

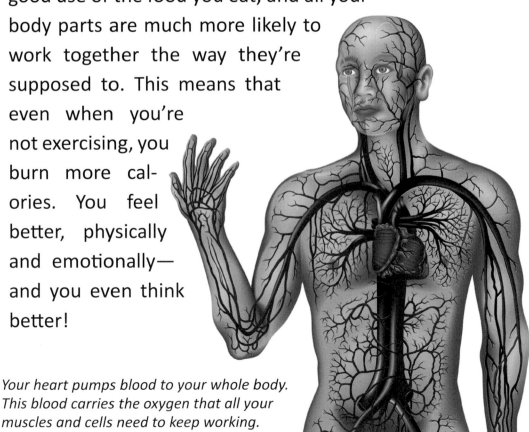

Your heart pumps blood to your whole body. This blood carries the oxygen that all your muscles and cells need to keep working.

EXERCISE AND YOUR HEART

You have big muscles in your arms and legs, and these get stronger when you exercise—but probably the most important muscle in your body is your heart. And it also gets stronger when you exercise.

Your heart works hard, pumping blood every day of your life. The blood carries oxygen to all the tiny cells in your body. The heart's job is what keeps you alive. Without oxygen, your cells would die. You would not be able to move or talk or think.

Your heart does this important job day after day, year after year, throughout your entire life. And when you exercise regularly, you help your heart do its job better— and odds are you will live longer.

The kind of exercise that is best for your heart is called aerobic exercise. "Aerobic" is a word that means "with air," and this kind of exercise means your body needs more oxygen than usual. You will breath faster, and your heart will beat faster, pumping oxygen-carrying blood to all your cells. If you give your heart this kind of workout a

DID YOU KNOW?

Here are some good aerobic exercises:

swimming
running
walking quickly
basketball
soccer
biking
jumping rope
roller blading
dancing

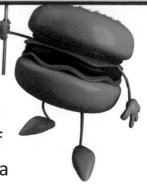

few times every week, your heart will get even better at its job, delivering oxygen to all the parts of your body.

EXERCISE AND YOUR OTHER MUSCLES

Aerobic exercises are good for your heart, but another kind of exercise is better at making your muscles stronger. This kind of exercises doesn't make you breathe as fast when you're doing it, but it builds strength. By using your muscles to push or pull heavy weights, you can make them better able to do their job.

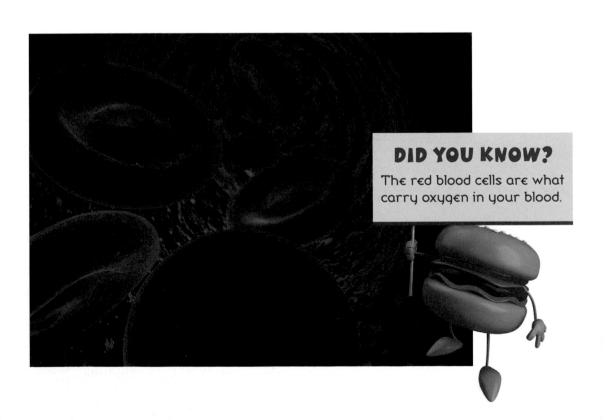

DID YOU KNOW?

The red blood cells are what carry oxygen in your blood.

But you don't have to use a weight machine to do this kind of exercise. Your body is a weight, too, and when you lift it or move it, you are using strength. This kind of workout can make muscles bigger and stronger.

DID YOU KNOW?

These exercises and activities will help you build strong muscles.

push-ups   pull-ups
rowing   running
bike riding

EXERCISE MAKES YOU FLEXIBLE

Can you touch your toes without bending your knees? Can you put one hand over your shoulder and the other behind your back—

Running is an excellent form of aerobic exercise—it makes you breathe harder and your heart beat faster.

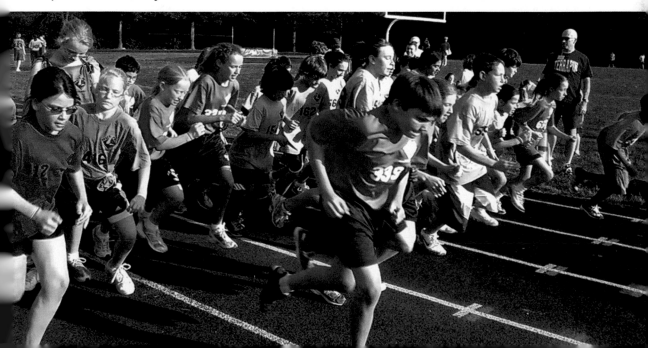

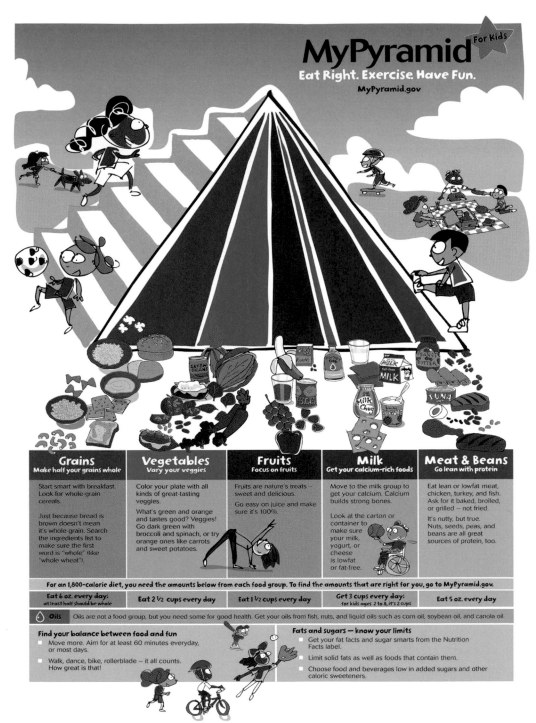

Exercise is important, and so is fueling your muscles with the right foods. The USDA MyPyramid gives suggestions for a healthy diet and exercise program.

and then connect your two hands? If you can, then you're flexible.

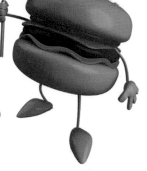

DID YOU KNOW?

Fewer than 1 out of every 4 children spend at least half an hour a day doing any sort of physical activity.

Being flexible means your muscles have full range of motion. You can move your arms and legs freely without feeling tightness or pain. Most children are fairly flexible, but as you get older, sometimes you lose some of your flexibility. Exercise can help you keep your body feeling young and flexible.

EXERCISE IS GOOD FOR YOUR BRAIN

Stretching before and after exercise can make your muscles more flexible and help prevent injuries.

You probably knew that exercise was good for your body. But did you know that exercise also helps you think better? Moving makes you breathe faster and your heart beat faster—and when you do, more blood flows to your brain. This means you can think more quickly and clearly.

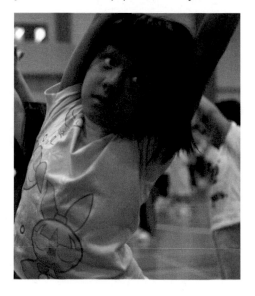

Scientists have found that exercise actually improves our memories. Regular exercise helps you learn more easily and think things through faster. It helps you concentrate. So if you want to be a better student, exercise!

EXERCISE MAKES YOU FEEL GOOD

It feels good to have a strong, flexible body that is able to have fun playing games and sports. But you don't have to be an athlete to enjoy exercise. Everyone feels better with a body that's strong and healthy.

Exercise also makes you feel happier because it causes your body to send chemicals called endorphins into your bloodstream. These chemicals improve your mood.

If you exercise regularly, you're less likely to feel sad and discouraged for very long. Life can be hard sometimes, and everyone gets upset—but exercise helps you cope with life's challenges. It releases some of the stress and tension that everyone feels sometimes.

That's why you need to make it a habit!

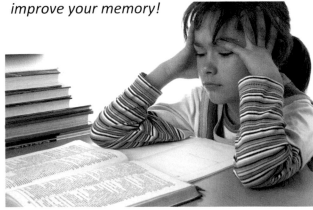

Do you have trouble with your homework? Getting more exercise might help—exercise can help your brain work better and even improve your memory!

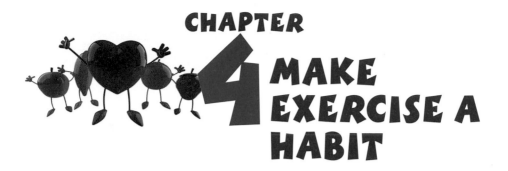

CHAPTER 4
MAKE EXERCISE A HABIT

Maybe you like sports. If you do, sports are a great way to get the exercise you need to be healthy. Play as much basketball, softball, soccer, hockey, lacrosse, or tennis as you can.

But maybe you DON'T like sports. That's okay too. But you still need to exercise regularly. You don't have to be an athlete to find ways to move your body.

Exercise should be fun. So pick something you genuinely enjoy doing. You'll be more likely to make exercise a habit if you like what you're doing.

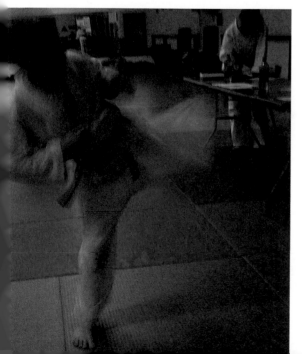

If you haven't been moving around much lately, start out slowly. Don't overdo it! It will be harder to stick with an exercise program if you make yourself tired and sore at the very beginning.

Baseball or football not your thing? Try some thing different like karate.

MAKING AN EXERCISE PLAN

Here are some suggestions that might help you make exercise a habit:

• Talk to your parents first. Explain why exercise is so important, and get their permission for whatever forms of exercise you choose to do. If you'll need rides or if your exercise schedule is going to cut into your parents' lives in some way, make sure you have their support.

• Encourage your family to exercise with you. Maybe your family could get a membership at a health club or the YMCA. Choose more active outings for family days together—hiking instead of going to a movie, for example, or swimming instead of staying home and watching television.

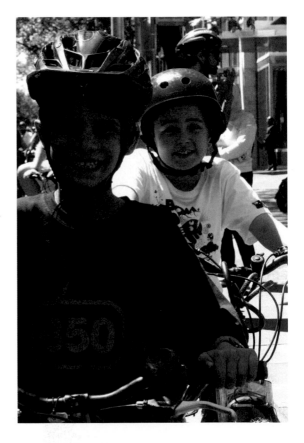

A bike ride with a friend will be good exercise and the friend will help keep it fun! Remember to always wear a helmet when riding your bike.

- Use the buddy system. If you have a friend who will exercise with you, you'll have more fun, and you'll be more likely to stick with it.

- Keep an exercise diary. Write down the days you exercise, the distance or length of time of your workout, and how you feel after each session.

- Don't push yourself too hard. You should be able to talk while you're exercising. If you can't, because you're breathing too hard, than you need to slow down your pace a little. Build your strength gradually.

Take a hike! Make sure you are safe—choose a trail everyone in the family can handle, bring a trail map or GPS, check the weather, bring sunscreen and bug spray, wear good shoes, and bring plenty of water and some snacks.

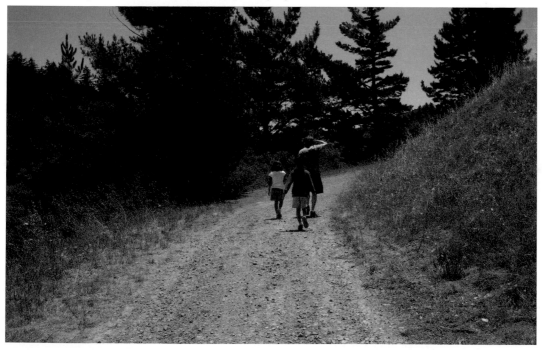

- If you miss a day, plan a make-up day. Don't double your exercise time during your next session. If you do, you're more likely to get too tired—if you're too tired, exercising won't seem like as much fun—and if you don't think exercise is fun, you're not as likely to keep doing it!

- If your form of exercise needs good weather, have a back-up indoor exercise plan for rainy days.

- Try something new. Take lessons to learn a new sport.

- Do different things different days, so you won't get bored. Take a walk one day, for example, go swimming the next, and then go for a bike ride on the weekend

- Try not to compare yourself with others. Having a strong healthy body doesn't mean you have to be a skilled athlete or win prizes. Being physically fit is about being in the best shape possible for YOU, regardless of how that compares with others.

DID YOU KNOW?

The National Association for Sports and Physical Education recommends that school-age kids:

- get 1 hour or more of moderate and vigorous physical activity on most or all days.

- also participate in several periods of physical activity of 15 minutes or more each day.

- avoid being inactive for 2 hours or more.

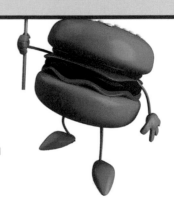

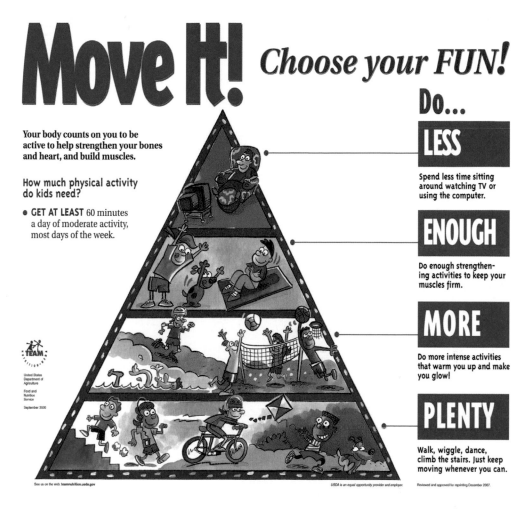

Move It!

Choose your FUN!

Do...

Your body counts on you to be active to help strengthen your bones and heart, and build muscles.

How much physical activity do kids need?

- **GET AT LEAST** 60 minutes a day of moderate activity, most days of the week.

LESS

Spend less time sitting around watching TV or using the computer.

ENOUGH

Do enough strengthening activities to keep your muscles firm.

MORE

Do more intense activities that warm you up and make you glow!

PLENTY

Walk, wiggle, dance, climb the stairs. Just keep moving whenever you can.

There are many choices when it comes to exercise—find the things you like and keep doing them!

- Be ready to change your exercise plan when needed. Any time there's a change in your family's routine, that will probably mean you have to build exercise back into your life all over again. For instance, if your mom starts a new job, she may not be able to pick you up anymore after basketball practice. Or when school lets out for the summer, you may finder it harder to keep up with your exercise program, even though you have more time. That's only normal. It just means you have to find new ways to build exercise back into your life again.

• Don't give up! Sometimes you won't feel like exercising and you'll just flop down and watch some TV instead. Don't feel angry with yourself—and don't get discouraged and drop your exercise plan altogether. Just get yourself going the next time. The more you exercise, the easier it will get—and the more it will become a habit for you.

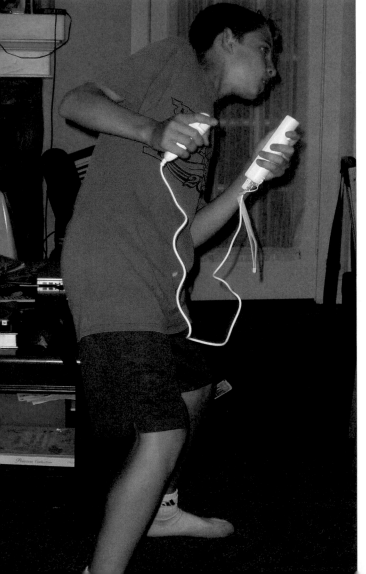

If you play video games, try and do something more active than just sitting on the couch.

GET PHYSICAL!

Here are some suggestions for ways you could build exercise into your life:

- Walk. Instead of asking your parents for a ride, use your own two feet whenever you can (or ride your bike). Not only will your body thank you but so will Planet Earth, since the more people don't rely on cars, the less air pollution there will be.
- Take the stairs. If you live in an apartment building or anytime you visit a building with elevators, don't push the elevator buttons. Instead, head for the stairwell and climb. Climbing stairs is a great workout.
- Try in-line skating. It's a fun, fast, easy-to-learn way to have a good time with your friends. Just remember to wear safety gear—a helmet and knee, wrist, and elbow pads.
- Walk the dog. And if you don't have a dog, volunteer to walk a neighbor's dog.

DID YOU KNOW?

When you're exercising, your body needs more water. You'll be able to exercise longer and stay healthier in the process if you take a break every now and then to drink plenty of water.

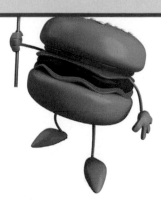

- Bike. (And don't forget to wear a helmet.)
- Do chores for your parents and neighbors (and maybe earn a few dollars at the same time!). Mowing lawns, weeding gardens, shoveling snow, and raking leaves will all burn calories and use your muscles.
- Dance! You don't have to go to a dance to shake your body. Any time you're listening to music, move in time with the beat.
- Babysit. Little kids move fast! Chasing after them can be great exercise.
- Swim whenever you get a chance. Swimming, diving, and even playing Marco Polo are all great ways to get your body moving.
- Play one-on-one basketball. All you need is a hoop in the driveway. Challenge your mom or your dad, your brother or your sister. First person to 21 wins!
- Fly a kite. You'll end up running more than you might think.

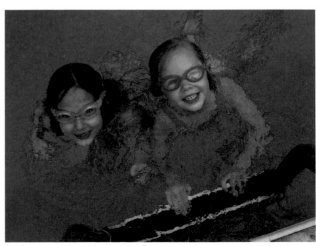

Swimming is fun and it is also good exercise. You can burn about 150–280 calories in an hour of just playing in the water, depending on your weight and how hard you play.

Exercise	Muscles Worked
Push-ups	Chest, shoulders, arms, abdominals
Sit-ups	Abdominals
Jumping Jacks	Calves (lower leg), inner/outer thigh, butt
Running	Calves, front/back thigh
Jumping rope	Calves, thighs, abdominals, shoulders, arms
Swimming	Nearly all major muscles
Dancing	Nearly all major muscles (depending on type of dance)
Walking	Arms, calves, front/back thigh, abdominals
Squats	Calves, front/back thigh, butt
Inline Skating	Inner/outer thigh, butt
Hula Hoop	Lower back, abdominals

SOURCE: American Council on Exercise

- Toss a Frisbee. Play catch with a friend—or with the dog. Either way, you'll be working your muscles.
- Hike. Ask your parents or grandparents to take you to a state park or other area where you can take a nature hike
- Play tag. It's a great aerobic activity.
- Play hopscotch.
- Have a hula hoop contest with a friend. See who can keep the hoop up the longest
- Learn to juggle
- Jump rope. It's not just for little girls. Did you know that boxers jump rope because it's such a good aerobic activity, plus it helps build coordination and quickness?
- Visit a zoo, amusement park, or museum with your family—and you'll end up doing lots of walking.

Anything that gets you moving can count as exercise!

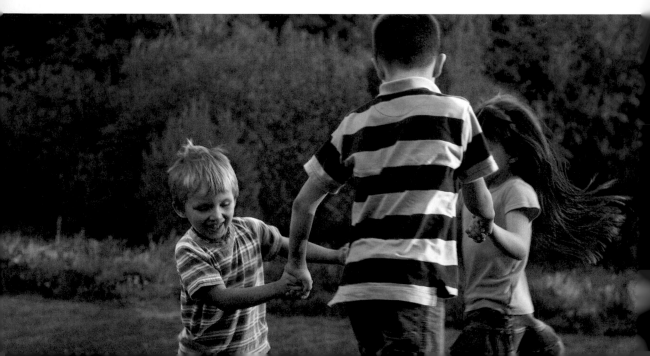

- Wash the car. It's good for your arm and shoulder muscles.
- Have a family walking contest. Every family member wears a pedometer once a week for a day—see who can take the most steps between breakfast and bedtime. Losers do the winner's chores the next day.
- Play badminton in the backyard. You'll do a lot of running as you chase after the birdie.

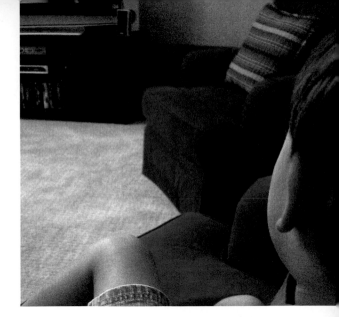

Watching some T.V. is ok, but limit it to less than two hours per day and don't snack while you watch. Instead of eating, add some exercise into those hours. Get up during commercials and dance, do jumping jacks, push-ups, or anything to get your heart rate up and your body moving.

- Have a water balloon fight.
- On a hot day, put on your bathing suit and run through the sprinkler.
- Give the dog a bath. The bigger the dog, the more exercise you'll get!
- Sign up for a charity walk-a-thon with your parent, grandparent, or other relative
- Do jumping jacks. There's nothing better for getting your heart and lungs working harder!
- Do push-ups or sit-ups—and build muscle strength.

- Put on an exercise video and get a good workout
- Learn to play golf—or caddy for someone else. You'll end up doing a lot of walking in the process.
- Play miniature golf—and you'll also do plenty of walking.
- Go bowling.
- Learn to twirl a baton.
- Take a class in martial arts. You'll get in shape—and learn other important skills in the process.
- Clean the house. Vacuuming, sweeping, dusting, and washing windows are all good exercise. Putting away clutter also involves plenty of bending and lifting and running up and down stairs.
- Ride a skateboard.
- Learn yoga, either at a class or from a video.
- Play touch football with your friends or family.
- Learn a new form of dance. Ballroom dancing, hip-hop, and ballet, jazz, or tap dancing are all excellent forms of aerobic exercise.
- Get a Wii.
- Ride an exercise bike or walk on a treadmill while watching television.

It really doesn't matter HOW you move—so long as you move!

READ MORE ABOUT IT

Ballard, Carol. *Keeping Fit: Body Systems.* Portsmouth, N.H.: Heinemann Educational Books, 2008.

Doeden, Matt. *Stay Fit! How You Can Get in Shape.* Minneapolis, Minn.: Lerner, 2009.

Gaesser, Glenn. *Big Fat Lies: The Truth About Your Weight and Your Health.* Carlsbad, Calif.: Gürze Books, 2002.

Gaff, Jackie. *Why Must I . . . Exercise?* London, U.K.: Cherrytree Books, 2005.

Kajander, Rebecca. *Be Fit, Be Strong, Be You*. Minneapolis, Minn.: Free Spirit Publishing, 2010.

Smithyman, Kathryn and Bobbie Kalman. *Active Kids.* New York: Crabtree Publishing, 2003.

Wallach, Marlene and Anna Palma. *My Life: A Guide to Health & Fitness.* New York: Aladdin, 2009.

FIND OUT MORE ON THE INTERNET

Activity Cards
www.bam.gov/sub_physicalactivity/physicalactivity_activitycards.html

Move It!
www.fns.usda.gov/tn/tnrockyrun/moveit.htm

MyPyramid Blast Off Game
www.mypyramid.gov/kids/kids_game.html

Small Step Kids
www.smallstep.gov/kids/html/games_and_activities.html

The websites listed on this page were active at the time of publication. The publisher is not responsible for websites that have changed their address or discontinued operation since the date of publication. The publisher will review and update the websites upon each reprint.

INDEX

PICTURE CREDITS

Creative Commons Attribution 2.0 Generic
   cambodia4kidsorg: pg. 35
   flattop341: pg. 40
   hoyasmeg: pg. 12
   lorda: pg. 38
   Tom@HK: pg. 31
   Uriel 1998: pg. 33
   zhurnaly: pg. 29
Creative Commons Attribution-Share Alike 2.0 Generic
   crimfants: pg. 21
   Extra Ketchup: pg. 25
   Ian Ransley Design and Illustration: pg. 16
   Takver: pg. 34

Food Standards Agency: pg. 8

Fotolia
   Cameraman: pg. 28
   Jacek Chabraszewski: pg. 32
   jedphoto: pg. 43
   Linda Macpherson: pg. 22
   Marzanna Syncerz: pg. 42
   Roman Dekan: pg. 26
   Vladislav Gajic: pg. 24

U.S.D.A.: pp 14, 30, 37

To the best knowledge of the publisher, all images not specifically credited are in the public domain. If any image has been inadvertently uncredited, please notify Harding House Publishing Service, 220 Front Street, Vestal, New York 13850, so that credit can be given in future printings.

Westfield Memorial Library
Westfield, New Jersey

ABOUT THE AUTHOR

Jamie Hunt is a certified teacher who has taught health to children from eleven to thirteen years old. She has worked with many publishers on a number of health-related books for young people. She lives in New York State.

WESTFIELD MEMORIAL LIBRARY

3 9550 00465 4173

Westfield Memorial Library
Westfield, New Jersey

J 613.7 Hun
Hunt, Jamie.
Getting stronger, getting fit

OCT 11